THE COMPLETE
NO POINT
WEIGHT LOSS
COOKBOOK

100+ No-Stress and Delicious Recipes to gain energy and lose weight without counting calories

BY
KATHERINE HOLT

Copyright © 2024 Katherine

All rights reserved. No part of this publication may be reproduced, distributed, or transmitted in any form or by any means, including photocopying, recording, or other electronic or mechanical methods, without the prior written permission of the publisher, except in the case of brief quotations embodied in critical reviews and certain other noncommercial uses permitted by copyright law.

INTRODUCTION 4

How to Use This Cookbook 6
Stocking Your Kitchen: Essentials for No Point Cooking 8
Understanding Key Ingredients 11
Tips for Meal Planning and Preparation 16
Smart Cooking Strategies 18

QUICK & EASY BREAKFASTS 20

Berry Bliss Smoothie Bowl 20
Overnight Chia Pudding 21
Veggie-Packed Omelette 21
Quinoa Breakfast Bowl 22
Greek Yogurt Parfait 23
Avocado Toast with Poached Egg 25
Peanut Butter Banana Oatmeal 25
Spinach and Feta Breakfast Wrap 26
Spinach and Feta Breakfast Wrap 27
Sweet Potato and Black Bean Breakfast Hash 28

SNACKS AND APPETIZERS 29

Baked Zucchini Chips 30
Hummus and Veggie Platter 30
Greek Yogurt and Cucumber Bites 31
Spicy Roasted Chickpeas 32
Guacamole with Baked Pita Chips 33
Caprese Skewers 34
Almond Butter Apple Slices 36
Edamame with Sea Salt 37
Avocado Deviled Eggs 38
Stuffed Mini Bell Peppers 39
Grilled Chicken Salad with Avocado and Mango 40

QUINOA AND BLACK BEAN STUFFED BELL PEPPERS	41
QUINOA AND BLACK BEAN STUFFED BELL PEPPERS	42
TURKEY AND AVOCADO LETTUCE WRAPS	43
VEGGIE-PACKED QUINOA BOWL	44

DINNER DELIGHTS 45

LEMON HERB BAKED COD WITH ASPARAGUS	45
SPAGHETTI SQUASH WITH TOMATO BASIL SAUCE	46
ONE-PAN BALSAMIC CHICKEN AND VEGETABLES	47
LENTIL AND VEGETABLE STIR-FRY	48

DESSERTS 49

CHOCOLATE AVOCADO MOUSSE	49
BAKED CINNAMON APPLES	50
BERRY CHIA PUDDING	51
COCONUT LIME ENERGY BITES	52
BAKED PEARS WITH WALNUTS AND HONEY	53
FROZEN BANANA BITES	54
GREEN DETOX SMOOTHIE	55
ICED HERBAL TEA WITH CITRUS	56
CUCUMBER MINT INFUSED WATER	57
ALMOND JOY SMOOTHIE	58
TURMERIC GINGER LATTE	59
WATERMELON BASIL COOLER	60

MEAL PLANS AND TIPS 61

TWO-WEEK NO POINT MEAL PLAN	61
HOW TO CUSTOMIZE RECIPES FOR DIETARY NEEDS	68

INTRODUCTION

The Philosophy Behind No Point Weight Loss

Welcome to "The Complete No Point Weight Loss Cookbook"! I'm thrilled to have you join me on this journey towards a healthier, more vibrant you. In this introduction, I want to share the philosophy behind the No Point Weight Loss approach. It's not just about shedding pounds—it's about gaining energy, feeling great, and enjoying delicious, stress-free meals.

The first thing you should know is that No Point Weight Loss focuses on simplicity. Forget about calculating calories, managing points, and meticulously measuring each component. This strategy is intended to reduce the stress associated with eating well. By focusing on full, nutrient-dense foods and responding to your body's natural hunger cues, you can accomplish long-term weight loss and better health without the stress of traditional dieting.

This attitude is based on a commitment to full, natural foods. Foods that are as close to their natural state as possible include fresh vegetables, fruits, lean proteins, whole grains, and healthy fats. Prioritizing these foods ensures that your body receives the nutrients it requires to function efficiently. This is not about scarcity; it is about abundance and diversity. You will learn how wonderful and satisfying genuine food can be.

Another important aspect of No Point Weight Loss is equilibrium. A well-balanced diet with a variety of macronutrients (carbohydrates, proteins, and fats) is essential. Each of these is essential for keeping your body stimulated and your metabolism functioning properly. I'll show you how to prepare balanced meals that are both nutritious and tasty.

Mindful eating is an effective tool in this process. This entails paying attention to what you eat and how it makes you feel. Are you eating for hunger or out of habit? Are you enjoying your meal or just mechanically munching? Being present at meals allows you to better understand your body's requirements and make healthy choices more easily.

Finally, the No Point Weight Loss concept emphasizes eliminating stress and guilt from the equation. Food should bring delight and sustenance, not cause concern. It's alright to indulge in a treat every now and then! It's about general habits and making healthier choices the majority of the time. This balanced approach assures that you can keep to it in the long run.

Don't forget that this is a trip, not a goal. There will be good times and bad times, which is normal. That's not the goal; the goal is growth. Remember to enjoy your wins, grow from your failures, and keep going. I'll be here with ideas, tips, and support every step of the way.

Welcome to the tasty and easy world of No Point Weight Loss! Let's dive in together. Wishing you health and happiness!

How to Use This Cookbook

There are parts in this cookbook that make it easy to find what you're looking for. We start with breakfasts to give you energy for the day, then move on to snacks and starters that you can eat without feeling guilty, and finally we get to lunches and dinners that will fill you up. There are also areas for drinks to cool you down, sides and salads to go with your main courses, and desserts and sweets to finish.

Understanding the Recipes

Each recipe is crafted with the No Point Weight Loss philosophy in mind. You'll find:

- **Ingredient Lists**: These are straightforward and use whole, natural foods. Ingredients are easy to find at your local grocery store.

- **Step-by-Step Instructions**: Detailed and easy-to-follow steps ensure you can prepare each dish with confidence, even if you're new to cooking.

- **Nutritional Information**: While we don't focus on calorie counting, I provide insights into the nutritional benefits of key ingredients, helping you understand how they support your health and weight loss goals.

Meal Planning and Prep Tips

To make your journey even easier, I've included tips on meal planning and preparation. At the end of the book, you'll find a sample weekly meal plan to help you get started. Meal prep tips are sprinkled throughout the book, offering advice on how to save time in the kitchen and ensure you always have healthy options on hand.

Flexibility and Customization

One of the best things about this cookbook is its flexibility. Many recipes are easily customizable to suit your tastes and dietary needs. I provide suggestions for ingredient swaps and additions, so you can make each dish your own. Whether you're vegetarian, gluten-free, or just looking to mix things up, there's something here for you.

Enjoy the Journey

Most importantly, have fun! Cooking should be a joyful and creative process. Don't be afraid to experiment with flavors and techniques. This is your journey to better health, and I'm here to support you every step of the way.

Stocking Your Kitchen: Essentials for No Point Cooking

A well-stocked kitchen is important if you want to get the most out of this cookbook and make easy, tasty, and healthy meals. Here is a list of the most important things you'll need to begin.

Fresh Produce

Vegetables: Fill your fridge with a variety of colorful vegetables. Think leafy greens like spinach and kale, cruciferous veggies like broccoli and cauliflower, and versatile staples like bell peppers, carrots, and zucchini. These are the foundation of many nutritious meals.

Fruits: Keep a mix of fresh fruits on hand for snacking, smoothies, and desserts. Berries, apples, bananas, and citrus fruits are all great choices.

Pantry Staples

Whole Grains: Stock up on quinoa, brown rice, whole wheat pasta, and oats. These grains are packed with fiber and essential nutrients, providing lasting energy.

Legumes: Beans, lentils, and chickpeas are excellent sources of plant-based protein and fiber. They're perfect for soups, stews, and salads.

Nuts and Seeds: Almonds, walnuts, chia seeds, and flaxseeds are nutrient-dense additions to many dishes. They're great for snacking, adding to salads, or blending into smoothies.

Healthy Oils: Olive oil, coconut oil, and avocado oil are all great for cooking and dressings. These oils provide healthy fats that are essential for your body.

Proteins

Lean Meats: Skinless chicken breasts, turkey, and lean cuts of beef are good sources of protein.

Seafood: Salmon, tuna, and shrimp are not only rich in protein but also provide healthy omega-3 fatty acids.

Plant-Based Proteins: Tofu, tempeh, and edamame are excellent for those following a vegetarian or vegan diet.

Dairy and Alternatives

Dairy: Greek yogurt, cottage cheese, and milk are versatile ingredients for many recipes.

Alternatives: Almond milk, soy milk, and other plant-based milks can be used in place of dairy.

Spices and Herbs

Basic Spices: Salt, pepper, garlic powder, onion powder, paprika, and chili powder are essential for seasoning.

Herbs: Fresh or dried herbs like basil, oregano, thyme, and cilantro add flavor and depth to your dishes.

Specialty Spices: Turmeric, cumin, curry powder, and ginger can bring exciting flavors to your meals.

Condiments and Sauces

Vinegars: Apple cider vinegar, balsamic vinegar, and rice vinegar are great for dressings and marinades.

Soy Sauce or Tamari: Useful for Asian-inspired dishes.

Mustards: Dijon and whole grain mustard add tang and depth to recipes.

Nut Butters: Almond butter and peanut butter are excellent for snacks and adding creaminess to sauces.

Kitchen Tools

Basic Utensils: A good set of knives, cutting boards, measuring cups and spoons, and mixing bowls are essential.

Pots and Pans: A variety of pots, pans, and baking dishes will allow you to cook a wide range of recipes.

Blender or Food Processor: Great for making smoothies, soups, and sauces.

Slow Cooker or Instant Pot: These appliances can save you time and make meal prep easier.

Preparing for Success

Having a well-stocked kitchen sets you up for success. When you have the right ingredients and tools at your fingertips, cooking healthy meals becomes easier and more enjoyable. Remember, the goal is to make your kitchen a place of creativity and nourishment.

Understanding Key Ingredients

As we start this cooking adventure together, it's important to know what the main things are that will make you successful. There are tasty and healthy recipes in this cookbook that are built around these items. Let's look more closely at what makes them unique and how they can help you reach your health and weight loss goals.

Fresh Produce

Leafy Greens: Spinach, kale, and Swiss chard are packed with vitamins A, C, and K, as well as fiber and antioxidants. They're low in calories and incredibly versatile, perfect for salads, smoothies, and stir-fries.

Cruciferous Vegetables: Broccoli, cauliflower, Brussels sprouts, and cabbage are known for their cancer-fighting properties. They're high in fiber, which helps you feel full longer, and rich in vitamins and minerals.

Colorful Veggies: Bell peppers, carrots, tomatoes, and beets are not only visually appealing but also loaded with nutrients like beta-carotene, vitamin C, and potassium. These vegetables add flavor, texture, and essential nutrients to your meals.

Fruits

Berries: Strawberries, blueberries, raspberries, and blackberries are antioxidant powerhouses. They're low in calories but high in fiber and vitamins, making them perfect for snacks, desserts, and smoothies.

Citrus Fruits: Oranges, lemons, limes, and grapefruits are excellent sources of vitamin C and fiber. They add a refreshing zing to salads, marinades, and drinks.

Bananas and Apples: These fruits are easy to find and incredibly versatile. They provide a good balance of natural sugars, fiber, and essential vitamins.

Whole Grains

Quinoa: This ancient grain is a complete protein, meaning it contains all nine essential amino acids. It's also high in fiber, iron, and magnesium, making it a fantastic base for salads, bowls, and side dishes.

Brown Rice: A whole grain that retains its bran and germ, brown rice is higher in fiber and nutrients than white rice. It's a great staple for a variety of dishes.

Oats: Rich in fiber and protein, oats are a wonderful breakfast option. They help regulate blood sugar levels and keep you feeling full longer.

Legumes

Beans: Black beans, kidney beans, and pinto beans are excellent sources of plant-based protein and fiber. They're versatile and can be used in soups, stews, salads, and even baked goods.

Lentils: These tiny legumes are packed with protein, fiber, iron, and folate. They cook quickly and are perfect for soups, salads, and casseroles.

Chickpeas: Also known as garbanzo beans, chickpeas are rich in protein, fiber, and essential vitamins. They're great in salads, hummus, and roasted for a crunchy snack.

Healthy Fats

Avocados: Full of heart-healthy monounsaturated fats, avocados are also rich in fiber, potassium, and vitamins C, E, and K. They add creaminess to dishes without the need for unhealthy fats.

Nuts and Seeds: Almonds, walnuts, chia seeds, and flaxseeds provide healthy fats, protein, and fiber. They're perfect for snacking, adding to salads, or blending into smoothies.

Olive Oil: A staple in healthy cooking, olive oil is rich in monounsaturated fats and antioxidants. Use it for sautéing, roasting, and dressing salads.

Proteins

Lean Meats: Skinless chicken breast, turkey, and lean cuts of beef are excellent sources of protein without excess fat. They're great for building muscle and keeping you satisfied.

Seafood: Salmon, tuna, and shrimp are high in protein and omega-3 fatty acids, which are essential for heart health. They're versatile and can be grilled, baked, or added to salads.

Plant-Based Proteins: Tofu, tempeh, and edamame are excellent sources of protein for vegetarians and vegans. They're versatile and can be used in a variety of dishes.

Dairy and Alternatives

Greek Yogurt: High in protein and probiotics, Greek yogurt is great for digestion and can be used in smoothies, dressings, and as a substitute for sour cream.

Milk and Alternatives: Whether you choose dairy milk or plant-based alternatives like almond or soy milk, these provide calcium and vitamin D, essential for bone health.

Spices and Herbs

Basic Spices: Salt, pepper, garlic powder, and onion powder are essential for flavoring your dishes. They're the backbone of any good seasoning blend.

Herbs: Fresh or dried, herbs like basil, oregano, thyme, and cilantro add flavor without extra calories. They also provide antioxidants and other health benefits.

Tips for Meal Planning and Preparation

For the No Point Weight Loss plan to work, you need to plan and prepare your meals ahead of time. You can always have healthy, tasty meals ready to go if you plan and prepare them ahead of time. This will help you stay on track and lower your stress. Here are some useful tips to help you plan and make meals like a pro.

Plan Your Week

Set Aside Time: Choose a specific day each week to plan your meals. This could be a weekend day when you have a bit more free time.

Create a Weekly Menu: Write down what you'll have for breakfast, lunch, dinner, and snacks each day. This helps you stay organized and ensures you're eating a variety of foods.

Balance Your Meals: Make sure each meal includes a mix of protein, healthy fats, and whole grains, along with plenty of vegetables and fruits.

Make a Shopping List

Check Your Pantry: Before you head to the store, see what you already have on hand. This prevents buying duplicates and helps use up what you already have.

Organize by Category: Write your shopping list by category (produce, dairy, grains, etc.) to make your shopping trip more efficient.

Stick to the List: Avoid impulse buys by sticking to your list. This helps you stay focused on your health goals and budget.

Batch Cooking

Cook in Bulk: Prepare large batches of grains, legumes, and proteins that can be used in multiple meals throughout the week. For example, cook a big pot of quinoa or brown rice, or bake several chicken breasts.

Chop Once, Use Multiple Times: Chop a variety of vegetables at once and store them in airtight containers. This makes it easy to add veggies to any meal.

Freeze for Later: Make double portions of soups, stews, and casseroles and freeze half for later. This is perfect for those days when you don't have time to cook from scratch.

Pre-Portion Meals

Use Containers: Invest in a set of good quality, airtight containers. Portion out your meals and snacks into these containers so they're ready to grab and go.

Label Everything: Label your containers with the contents and date. This helps you keep track of what needs to be eaten first and prevents waste.

Prepare Snacks: Have healthy snacks ready, like sliced veggies, hummus, and fruit. This makes it easier to choose healthy options when hunger strikes.

Smart Cooking Strategies

One-Pot Meals: Save time on cleanup by making one-pot meals like soups, stews, and casseroles. These meals are not only convenient but also packed with flavor.

Sheet Pan Dinners: Cook an entire meal on one sheet pan. Simply toss your protein and veggies with some olive oil and seasoning, spread them out on a sheet pan, and roast in the oven.

Use a Slow Cooker or Instant Pot: These appliances can be lifesavers for busy weeks. Throw your ingredients in before you leave for work, and come home to a hot, ready-to-eat meal.

Keep It Simple

Focus on Simplicity: You don't need to prepare elaborate meals every day. Simple, wholesome dishes are often the best. Think grilled chicken with a side of roasted veggies or a hearty salad with beans and quinoa.

Mix and Match: Use the same base ingredients in different ways to keep things interesting. For example, grilled chicken can be used in salads, wraps, or stir-fries.

Theme Nights: To make planning easier, designate each night of the week with a theme, such as Meatless Monday, Taco Tuesday, or Stir-Fry Friday.

Stay Flexible

Allow for Flexibility: Life happens, and sometimes you'll need to adjust your plans. Keep a few easy, healthy meal options on hand for those days when things don't go as planned.

Listen to Your Body: Be open to adjusting your meals based on how you're feeling. If you're not very hungry one evening, it's okay to have a lighter meal or save a planned meal for the next day.

QUICK & EASY BREAKFASTS

Berry Bliss Smoothie Bowl

INGREDIENTS	DIRECTIONS
- 1 cup unsweetened almond milk - 1 cup frozen mixed berries - 1 banana, sliced - 1 tablespoon chia seeds - 1 tablespoon almond butter - 1/2 cup Greek yogurt - 1/4 cup granola - Fresh berries and sliced banana, for topping	1. In a blender, combine the almond milk, frozen mixed berries, banana, chia seeds, almond butter, and Greek yogurt. Blend until smooth and creamy. 2. Pour the smoothie into a bowl. 3. Top with granola, fresh berries, and sliced banana. 4. Serve immediately and enjoy! **Prep Time:** 10 minutes **Cooking Time:** 0 minutes **Servings:** 2

Why I Recommend This Recipe: This Berry Bliss Smoothie Bowl is a powerhouse of nutrients, perfect for a refreshing and energizing start to your day. The combination of fruits, chia seeds, and Greek yogurt provides fiber, protein, and healthy fats, helping you feel full and satisfied without counting calories.

Overnight Chia Pudding

INGREDIENTS	DIRECTIONS
- 1/4 cup chia seeds - 1 cup unsweetened almond milk - 1 teaspoon vanilla extract - 1 tablespoon maple syrup (optional) - Fresh fruit and nuts for topping	1. In a medium bowl, combine the chia seeds, almond milk, vanilla extract, and maple syrup if using. Stir well to combine. 2. Cover and refrigerate overnight or for at least 4 hours until the mixture thickens. 3. In the morning, stir the pudding and add more almond milk if needed to achieve your desired consistency. 4. Top with fresh fruit and nuts before serving. **Prep Time:** 5 minutes **Cooking Time:** 0 minutes (4 hours chilling) **Servings:** 2

Why I Recommend This Recipe: Overnight Chia Pudding is a no-stress, make-ahead breakfast that's rich in omega-3 fatty acids, fiber, and protein. It's perfect for busy mornings when you need a quick and nutritious meal that supports your weight loss goals.

Veggie-Packed Omelette

INGREDIENTS

- 3 large eggs
- 1/4 cup diced bell peppers
- 1/4 cup diced tomatoes
- 1/4 cup chopped spinach
- 1/4 cup diced onions
- 1 tablespoon olive oil
- Salt and pepper to taste

DIRECTIONS

1. In a medium bowl, beat the eggs and season with salt and pepper.
2. Heat olive oil in a non-stick skillet over medium heat.
3. Add the bell peppers, tomatoes, spinach, and onions to the skillet. Sauté for 3-4 minutes until the vegetables are tender.
4. Pour the beaten eggs over the vegetables. Let cook without stirring until the edges start to set.
5. Gently lift the edges with a spatula, allowing the uncooked eggs to flow underneath. Continue until the omelette is mostly set but still slightly runny on top.
6. Fold the omelette in half and cook for another minute.
7. Slide the omelette onto a plate and serve immediately.

Prep Time: 10 minutes
Cooking Time: 10 minutes
Servings: 1

Why I Recommend This Recipe: This Veggie-Packed Omelette is a nutritious, protein-rich breakfast that's loaded with vitamins and minerals from the fresh vegetables. It's an easy way to start your day with a satisfying meal that supports your weight loss goals.

Quinoa Breakfast Bowl

INGREDIENTS	DIRECTIONS
- 1 cup cooked quinoa - 1/2 avocado, sliced - 1/2 cup cherry tomatoes, halved - 1/4 cup black beans, rinsed and drained - 1 large egg - 1 tablespoon olive oil - 1 tablespoon chopped fresh cilantro - Salt and pepper to taste	1. In a medium skillet, heat the olive oil over medium heat. 2. Crack the egg into the skillet and cook to your desired doneness (sunny-side up or over-easy). 3. In a bowl, layer the cooked quinoa, avocado slices, cherry tomatoes, and black beans. 4. Top with the cooked egg. 5. Sprinkle with chopped cilantro, salt, and pepper. 6. Serve immediately. **Prep Time:** 10 minutes **Cooking Time:** 5 minutes **Servings:** 1

Why I Recommend This Recipe: The Quinoa Breakfast Bowl is a balanced meal packed with protein, healthy fats, and fiber. It provides sustained energy to keep you full throughout the morning, making it a perfect choice for those aiming to lose weight without feeling deprived.

Greek Yogurt Parfait

INGREDIENTS

- 1 cup Greek yogurt
- 1/2 cup granola
- 1/2 cup mixed berries (strawberries, blueberries, raspberries)
- 1 tablespoon honey (optional)

DIRECTIONS

1. In a glass or bowl, layer half of the Greek yogurt.
2. Add a layer of mixed berries and granola.
3. Repeat with the remaining Greek yogurt, berries, and granola.
4. Drizzle with honey if using.
5. Serve immediately.

Prep Time: 5 minutes
Cooking Time: 0 minutes
Servings: 1

Why I Recommend This Recipe: This Greek Yogurt Parfait is a quick and easy breakfast option that's rich in protein and antioxidants. The combination of creamy yogurt, crunchy granola, and fresh berries makes it a satisfying and healthy start to your day, aligning perfectly with the no-stress, nutritious focus of the cookbook.

Avocado Toast with Poached Egg

INGREDIENTS

- 1 ripe avocado
- 2 slices whole grain bread
- 2 large eggs
- 1 tablespoon lemon juice
- Salt and pepper to taste
- Red pepper flakes (optional)
- Fresh herbs (optional, such as parsley or cilantro)

DIRECTIONS

- Toast the whole grain bread slices until golden brown.
- Cut the avocado in half, remove the pit, and scoop the flesh into a bowl. Mash with a fork and add lemon juice, salt, and pepper to taste.
- Spread the mashed avocado evenly over the toasted bread.
- Bring a pot of water to a gentle simmer and add a splash of vinegar (optional). Crack an egg into a small bowl, then gently slide it into the simmering water. Poach for about 3-4 minutes, or until the white is set but the yolk is still runny. Repeat with the second egg.
- Carefully remove the poached eggs with a slotted spoon and place one on each slice of avocado toast.
- Sprinkle with red pepper flakes and fresh herbs, if desired.
- Serve immediately.

Prep Time: 10 minutes
Cooking Time: 5 minutes
Servings: 2

Why I Recommend This Recipe: Avocado Toast with Poached Egg is a nutrient-dense breakfast packed with healthy fats, protein, and fiber. It's quick to prepare and keeps you full and energized, making it a fantastic choice for starting your day right.

Peanut Butter Banana Oatmeal

INGREDIENTS

- 1 cup rolled oats
- 2 cups water or unsweetened almond milk
- 1 ripe banana, sliced
- 2 tablespoons natural peanut butter
- 1 teaspoon cinnamon
- 1 tablespoon chia seeds (optional)
- Honey or maple syrup to taste (optional)

DIRECTIONS

1. In a medium saucepan, bring the water or almond milk to a boil.
2. Add the rolled oats and reduce the heat to a simmer. Cook, stirring occasionally, until the oats are soft and have absorbed most of the liquid, about 5 minutes.
3. Stir in the sliced banana, peanut butter, and cinnamon. Cook for another 2-3 minutes until heated through.
4. Remove from heat and stir in the chia seeds if using.
5. Serve in bowls, drizzling with honey or maple syrup if desired.

Prep Time: 5 minutes
Cooking Time: 10 minutes
Servings: 2

Why I Recommend This Recipe: Peanut Butter Banana Oatmeal is a warm, comforting breakfast that's rich in fiber, protein, and healthy fats. The combination of oats and chia seeds provides lasting energy, while the banana and peanut butter add natural sweetness and creaminess.

Spinach and Feta Breakfast Wrap

INGREDIENTS

- 2 whole wheat tortillas
- 4 large eggs
- 1 cup fresh spinach leaves
- 1/4 cup crumbled feta cheese
- 1 tablespoon olive oil
- Salt and pepper to taste
- Hot sauce (optional)

DIRECTIONS

1. In a medium bowl, whisk the eggs with salt and pepper.
2. Heat the olive oil in a non-stick skillet over medium heat. Add the spinach and cook until wilted, about 2 minutes.
3. Pour the eggs into the skillet and cook, stirring gently, until the eggs are scrambled and set.
4. Remove from heat and stir in the crumbled feta cheese.
5. Warm the tortillas in a dry skillet or microwave.
6. Divide the egg mixture between the two tortillas and wrap them up.
7. Serve immediately with hot sauce if desired.

Prep Time: 10 minutes
Cooking Time: 5 minutes
Servings: 2

Why I Recommend This Recipe: The Spinach and Feta Breakfast Wrap is a portable, protein-packed meal that's perfect for busy mornings. The fresh spinach adds a dose of vitamins, while the feta provides a tangy flavor boost. This wrap is easy to make and keeps you satisfied for hours.

Spinach and Feta Breakfast Wrap

INGREDIENTS

- 1 cup cottage cheese (low-fat or full-fat)
- 1/2 cup mixed fresh fruit (such as berries, pineapple, and melon)
- 1 tablespoon honey
- 1 tablespoon chopped nuts (such as almonds or walnuts)
- Fresh mint leaves (optional)

DIRECTIONS

1. Scoop the cottage cheese into a bowl.
2. Top with mixed fresh fruit.
3. Drizzle with honey.
4. Sprinkle with chopped nuts and garnish with fresh mint leaves if desired.
5. Serve immediately.

Prep Time: 5 minutes
Cooking Time: 0 minutes
Servings: 1

Why I Recommend This Recipe: Cottage Cheese and Fruit Bowl is a simple, refreshing breakfast that's high in protein and packed with vitamins and minerals. The combination of cottage cheese and fruit provides a balanced mix of nutrients to start your day on a healthy note.

Sweet Potato and Black Bean Breakfast Hash

INGREDIENTS

- 1 large sweet potato, peeled and diced
- 1/2 cup black beans, rinsed and drained
- 1 small onion, diced
- 1 red bell pepper, diced
- 2 tablespoons olive oil
- 1 teaspoon cumin
- 1 teaspoon paprika
- Salt and pepper to taste
- 2 large eggs
- Fresh cilantro, chopped (optional)

DIRECTIONS

1. Heat the olive oil in a large skillet over medium heat.
2. Add the diced sweet potato and cook for about 10 minutes, stirring occasionally, until tender and starting to brown.
3. Add the onion and red bell pepper to the skillet. Cook for another 5 minutes until the vegetables are softened.
4. Stir in the black beans, cumin, paprika, salt, and pepper. Cook for an additional 2-3 minutes until everything is heated through.
5. In a separate skillet, cook the eggs to your desired doneness (fried, scrambled, or poached).
6. Serve the sweet potato hash topped with the eggs and garnished with fresh cilantro if desired.

Prep Time: 10 minutes
Cooking Time: 15 minutes
Servings: 2

Why I Recommend This Recipe: Sweet Potato and Black Bean Breakfast Hash is a hearty, nutrient-dense meal that's perfect for starting your day with a boost of energy. The sweet potatoes provide complex carbohydrates and fiber, while the black beans and eggs add protein and healthy fats. This balanced breakfast keeps you full and satisfied, supporting your weight loss journey.

Snacks and Appetizers

Baked Zucchini Chips

INGREDIENTS

- 2 medium zucchinis
- 2 tablespoons olive oil
- 1/2 cup grated Parmesan cheese
- 1 teaspoon garlic powder
- 1 teaspoon paprika
- Salt and pepper to taste

DIRECTIONS

1. Preheat your oven to 425°F (220°C). Line a baking sheet with parchment paper.
2. Slice the zucchinis into thin rounds, about 1/8-inch thick.
3. In a large bowl, toss the zucchini slices with olive oil, Parmesan cheese, garlic powder, paprika, salt, and pepper until evenly coated.
4. Arrange the zucchini slices in a single layer on the prepared baking sheet.
5. Bake for 25-30 minutes, turning once halfway through, until the chips are golden and crispy.
6. Let cool for a few minutes before serving.

Prep Time: 10 minutes
Cooking Time: 25-30 minutes
Servings: 4

Why I Recommend This Recipe. Baked Zucchini Chips are a healthy, low-calorie alternative to traditional potato chips. They're packed with flavor and nutrients, making them a perfect snack to satisfy your cravings without derailing your weight loss efforts.

Hummus and Veggie Platter

INGREDIENTS

- 1 can (15 oz) chickpeas, drained and rinsed
- 1/4 cup tahini
- 1/4 cup fresh lemon juice
- 2 tablespoons olive oil
- 2 garlic cloves, minced
- 1/2 teaspoon cumin
- Salt to taste
- 2-3 tablespoons water (as needed)
- Fresh veggies (carrot sticks, cucumber slices, bell pepper strips, cherry tomatoes)

DIRECTIONS

1. In a food processor, combine the chickpeas, tahini, lemon juice, olive oil, garlic, cumin, and salt. Blend until smooth.
2. Add water, one tablespoon at a time, until the hummus reaches your desired consistency.
3. Transfer the hummus to a serving bowl.
4. Arrange the fresh veggies around the bowl of hummus.
5. Serve immediately or refrigerate until ready to serve.

Prep Time: 15 minutes
Cooking Time: 0 minutes
Servings: 6

Why I Recommend This Recipe: Hummus and Veggie Platter is a nutrient-dense, satisfying snack that's easy to prepare. The hummus provides protein and healthy fats, while the fresh veggies offer a variety of vitamins and minerals, making it an excellent choice for a balanced, no-point snack.

Greek Yogurt and Cucumber Bites

INGREDIENTS

- 1 large cucumber, sliced into rounds
- 1 cup Greek yogurt
- 1 tablespoon fresh dill, chopped
- 1 tablespoon fresh lemon juice
- 1 garlic clove, minced
- Salt and pepper to taste
- Fresh dill for garnish (optional)

DIRECTIONS

1. In a bowl, mix the Greek yogurt, chopped dill, lemon juice, minced garlic, salt, and pepper until well combined.
2. Place a small dollop of the yogurt mixture on each cucumber slice.
3. Garnish with a small sprig of fresh dill if desired.
4. Arrange on a platter and serve immediately.

Prep Time: 10 minutes
Cooking Time: 0 minutes
Servings: 4

Why I Recommend This Recipe: Greek Yogurt and Cucumber Bites are a refreshing, low-calorie snack that's high in protein and probiotics. They're quick to prepare and perfect for a light, satisfying bite that supports your weight loss goals.

Spicy Roasted Chickpeas

INGREDIENTS

- 1 can (15 oz) chickpeas, drained and rinsed
- 1 tablespoon olive oil
- 1 teaspoon smoked paprika
- 1/2 teaspoon cumin
- 1/2 teaspoon garlic powder
- 1/4 teaspoon cayenne pepper
- Salt to taste

DIRECTIONS

1. Preheat your oven to 400°F (200°C). Line a baking sheet with parchment paper.
2. Pat the chickpeas dry with a paper towel.
3. In a bowl, toss the chickpeas with olive oil, smoked paprika, cumin, garlic powder, cayenne pepper, and salt until evenly coated.
4. Spread the chickpeas in a single layer on the prepared baking sheet.
5. Roast for 25-30 minutes, shaking the pan halfway through, until the chickpeas are crispy and golden.
6. Let cool slightly before serving.

Prep Time: 10 minutes
Cooking Time: 25-30 minutes
Servings: 4

Why I Recommend This Recipe: Spicy Roasted Chickpeas are a crunchy, high-protein snack that's full of flavor and easy to make. They're a great alternative to unhealthy, processed snacks and help keep you full and satisfied between meals.

Guacamole with Baked Pita Chips

INGREDIENTS

- 3 ripe avocados
- 1 small red onion, finely diced
- 1 medium tomato, diced
- 1 jalapeño, seeded and minced
- 1/4 cup fresh cilantro, chopped
- 2 tablespoons fresh lime juice
- Salt and pepper to taste
- 4 whole wheat pitas
- 2 tablespoons olive oil
- 1 teaspoon garlic powder
- 1 teaspoon paprika

DIRECTIONS

1. Preheat your oven to 375°F (190°C). Line a baking sheet with parchment paper.
2. Cut the pitas into triangles and place them on the baking sheet.
3. Brush the pita triangles with olive oil and sprinkle with garlic powder and paprika.
4. Bake for 10-12 minutes, or until the pita chips are crispy and golden. Let cool.
5. Meanwhile, in a bowl, mash the avocados with a fork.
6. Add the diced red onion, tomato, jalapeño, cilantro, lime juice, salt, and pepper. Mix until well combined.
7. Serve the guacamole with the baked pita chips.

Prep Time: 15 minutes
Cooking Time: 10-12 minutes
Servings: 6

Why I Recommend This Recipe: Guacamole with Baked Pita Chips is a nutritious and delicious snack that's rich in healthy fats, fiber, and vitamins. The homemade pita chips are a healthier alternative to store-bought options, and the guacamole is bursting with fresh flavors, making it an ideal snack for weight loss and overall health.

Caprese Skewers

INGREDIENTS

- 1 pint cherry tomatoes
- 1 block fresh mozzarella cheese, cut into bite-sized cubes
- Fresh basil leaves
- 2 tablespoons balsamic glaze
- Salt and pepper to taste
- Wooden skewers or toothpicks

DIRECTIONS

1. Thread a cherry tomato, a piece of fresh basil, and a cube of mozzarella onto each skewer or toothpick. Repeat until all ingredients are used.
2. Arrange the skewers on a serving platter.
3. Drizzle with balsamic glaze and season with salt and pepper.
4. Serve immediately.

Prep Time: 10 minutes
Cooking Time: 0 minutes
Servings: 6

Why I Recommend This Recipe: Caprese Skewers are a light and refreshing snack that's easy to prepare and full of flavor. The combination of juicy tomatoes, creamy mozzarella, and aromatic basil makes for a satisfying, low-calorie snack that's perfect for any time of day.

Almond Butter Apple Slices

INGREDIENTS

- 2 large apples, cored and sliced
- 1/4 cup almond butter
- 2 tablespoons unsweetened coconut flakes
- 2 tablespoons chopped nuts (such as almonds or walnuts)
- 1 teaspoon ground cinnamon

DIRECTIONS

1. Arrange the apple slices on a serving platter.
2. Spread a small amount of almond butter on each apple slice.
3. Sprinkle with coconut flakes, chopped nuts, and ground cinnamon.
4. Serve immediately.

Prep Time: 5 minutes
Cooking Time: 0 minutes
Servings: 4

Why I Recommend This Recipe: Almond Butter Apple Slices are a nutritious and delicious snack that combines the sweetness of apples with the protein and healthy fats from almond butter. This snack is perfect for curbing hunger between meals and provides a balanced mix of nutrients.

Edamame with Sea Salt

INGREDIENTS

- 2 cups frozen edamame (soybeans) in pods
- 1 teaspoon sea salt
- 1 teaspoon sesame oil (optional)

DIRECTIONS

1. Bring a large pot of water to a boil. Add the frozen edamame and cook for 3-5 minutes, until tender.
2. Drain the edamame and transfer to a bowl.
3. Toss with sea salt and sesame oil, if using.
4. Serve immediately.

Prep Time: 5 minutes
Cooking Time: 5 minutes
Servings: 4

Why I Recommend This Recipe: Edamame with Sea Salt is a simple, high-protein snack that's easy to prepare and enjoy. Edamame is rich in fiber, protein, and essential nutrients, making it an excellent choice for a healthy, satisfying snack.

Avocado Deviled Eggs

INGREDIENTS

- 6 large eggs
- 1 ripe avocado
- 1 tablespoon lime juice
- 1 tablespoon chopped fresh cilantro
- 1 garlic clove, minced
- Salt and pepper to taste
- Paprika for garnish

DIRECTIONS

1. Place the eggs in a saucepan and cover with water. Bring to a boil, then reduce the heat and simmer for 10 minutes.
2. Remove the eggs from the hot water and cool in an ice bath. Peel the eggs and cut them in half lengthwise.
3. Scoop out the yolks and place them in a bowl.
4. Add the avocado, lime juice, cilantro, garlic, salt, and pepper to the yolks. Mash until smooth.
5. Spoon the avocado mixture into the egg whites.
6. Sprinkle with paprika and serve immediately.

Prep Time: 15 minutes
Cooking Time: 10 minutes
Servings: 12 halves

Why I Recommend This Recipe: Avocado Deviled Eggs are a creamy, protein-packed snack with healthy fats from the avocado. They're a great alternative to traditional deviled eggs and provide a satisfying, low-carb option that supports your weight loss goals.

Stuffed Mini Bell Peppers

INGREDIENTS

- 1 pound mini bell peppers, halved and seeded
- 1 cup quinoa, cooked
- 1/2 cup black beans, rinsed and drained
- 1/4 cup corn kernels
- 1/4 cup diced red onion
- 1/4 cup chopped fresh cilantro
- 1 tablespoon lime juice
- Salt and pepper to taste

DIRECTIONS

1. Preheat your oven to 375°F (190°C). Line a baking sheet with parchment paper.
2. In a bowl, combine the cooked quinoa, black beans, corn, red onion, cilantro, lime juice, salt, and pepper.
3. Spoon the quinoa mixture into the halved mini bell peppers.
4. Arrange the stuffed peppers on the prepared baking sheet.
5. Bake for 10-15 minutes, until the peppers are tender.
6. Serve immediately.

Prep Time: 15 minutes
Cooking Time: 10-15 minutes
Servings: 4

Why I Recommend This Recipe: Stuffed Mini Bell Peppers are a colorful, nutritious snack that's easy to make and packed with flavor. The quinoa and black beans provide protein and fiber, while the fresh veggies add a variety of vitamins and minerals. This snack is perfect for keeping you full and energized.

Grilled Chicken Salad with Avocado and Mango

INGREDIENTS

- 2 boneless, skinless chicken breasts
- 1 tablespoon olive oil
- Salt and pepper to taste
- 6 cups mixed greens (such as spinach, arugula, and romaine)
- 1 ripe avocado, sliced
- 1 ripe mango, diced
- 1/2 red onion, thinly sliced
- 1/4 cup chopped fresh cilantro
- 1/4 cup crumbled feta cheese (optional)
- 1/4 cup toasted pumpkin seeds

For the Dressing:
- 3 tablespoons olive oil
- 2 tablespoons fresh lime juice
- 1 tablespoon honey
- 1 teaspoon Dijon mustard
- Salt and pepper to taste

DIRECTIONS

- Preheat the grill to medium-high heat. Season the chicken breasts with olive oil, salt, and pepper.

- Grill the chicken for 6-7 minutes on each side, or until fully cooked and the internal temperature reaches 165°F (75°C). Let the chicken rest for a few minutes, then slice it thinly.

- In a small bowl, whisk together the dressing ingredients: olive oil, lime juice, honey, Dijon mustard, salt, and pepper.

- In a large bowl, combine the mixed greens, avocado, mango, red onion, cilantro, and feta cheese if using. Toss with the dressing until evenly coated.

- Top the salad with the sliced grilled chicken and toasted pumpkin seeds.

- Serve immediately.

Prep Time: 15 minutes

Cooking Time: 15 minutes

Servings: 4

Why I Recommend This Recipe: Grilled Chicken Salad with Avocado and Mango is a refreshing and protein-packed lunch that combines the lean protein of chicken with the healthy fats from avocado and the natural sweetness of mango. It's a perfect, nutrient-dense meal to keep you full and energized throughout the day without any calorie counting.

Quinoa and Black Bean Stuffed Bell Peppers

INGREDIENTS

- 4 large bell peppers, halved and seeded
- 1 cup quinoa, cooked
- 1 can (15 oz) black beans, rinsed and drained
- 1 cup corn kernels (fresh, frozen, or canned)
- 1 cup diced tomatoes
- 1/2 cup diced red onion
- 1/4 cup chopped fresh cilantro
- 1 tablespoon olive oil
- 1 teaspoon cumin
- 1 teaspoon chili powder
- Salt and pepper to taste
- 1/2 cup shredded cheddar cheese (optional)

DIRECTIONS

Instructions:

1. Preheat your oven to 375°F (190°C). Line a baking dish with parchment paper or lightly grease it.
2. In a large bowl, combine the cooked quinoa, black beans, corn, diced tomatoes, red onion, cilantro, olive oil, cumin, chili powder, salt, and pepper. Mix until well combined.
3. Stuff each bell pepper half with the quinoa mixture and place them in the prepared baking dish.
4. Cover the baking dish with aluminum foil and bake for 30 minutes.
5. If using, remove the foil and sprinkle the shredded cheddar cheese on top of each stuffed pepper. Bake for an additional 10 minutes, or until the cheese is melted and bubbly.
6. Remove from the oven and let cool slightly. Serve with lime wedges.

Prep Time: 20 minutes
Cooking Time: 40 minutes
Servings: 4

Why I Recommend This Recipe: Quinoa and Black Bean Stuffed Bell Peppers are a hearty and flavorful lunch option that's rich in protein, fiber, and essential nutrients. The combination of quinoa, black beans, and vegetables makes this dish both satisfying and nutritious, supporting your weight loss journey without the need for calorie counting.

Quinoa and Black Bean Stuffed Bell Peppers

INGREDIENTS

- 1 can (15 oz) chickpeas, drained and rinsed
- 1 cup cherry tomatoes, halved
- 1 cucumber, diced
- 1/2 red onion, finely chopped
- 1/4 cup Kalamata olives, pitted and sliced
- 1/4 cup crumbled feta cheese
- 2 tablespoons chopped fresh parsley
- 2 tablespoons chopped fresh mint (optional)
- 3 tablespoons olive oil
- 2 tablespoons red wine vinegar
- 1 teaspoon dried oregano
- Salt and pepper to taste

DIRECTIONS

1. In a large bowl, combine the chickpeas, cherry tomatoes, cucumber, red onion, Kalamata olives, feta cheese, parsley, and mint if using.
2. In a small bowl, whisk together the olive oil, red wine vinegar, dried oregano, salt, and pepper.
3. Pour the dressing over the salad and toss until all the ingredients are evenly coated.
4. Let the salad sit for at least 10 minutes to allow the flavors to meld.
5. Serve immediately or refrigerate until ready to eat.

Prep Time: 15 minutes
Cooking Time: 0 minutes
Servings: 4

Why I Recommend This Recipe: Mediterranean Chickpea Salad is a light yet filling lunch that's packed with plant-based protein, fiber, and a variety of vitamins and minerals. The fresh vegetables and herbs provide a burst of flavor, making this salad a satisfying and nutritious choice for weight loss.

Turkey and Avocado Lettuce Wraps

INGREDIENTS

- 1 pound ground turkey
- 1 tablespoon olive oil
- 1 small onion, finely chopped
- 2 garlic cloves, minced
- 1 teaspoon ground cumin
- 1 teaspoon paprika
- Salt and pepper to taste
- 1 head of romaine or butter lettuce, leaves separated and washed
- 1 ripe avocado, sliced
- 1/2 cup diced tomatoes
- 1/4 cup shredded carrot
- 1/4 cup chopped fresh cilantro

DIRECTIONS

1. Heat the olive oil in a large skillet over medium heat. Add the onion and garlic, and cook until softened, about 3 minutes.
2. Add the ground turkey, cumin, paprika, salt, and pepper. Cook, breaking up the meat with a spoon, until the turkey is browned and cooked through, about 7-10 minutes.
3. Remove from heat and let cool slightly.
4. To assemble the wraps, place a few slices of avocado, a spoonful of the turkey mixture, diced tomatoes, shredded carrot, and cilantro onto each lettuce leaf.
5. Serve immediately with lime wedges on the side for squeezing over the wraps.

Prep Time: 15 minutes
Cooking Time: 10 minutes
Servings: 4

Why I Recommend This Recipe: Turkey and Avocado Lettuce Wraps are a delicious, low-carb lunch option that's high in protein and healthy fats. The lettuce wraps are light and refreshing, while the ground turkey and avocado provide a satisfying and nutrient-dense filling. This meal is perfect for maintaining energy levels and supporting weight loss without counting calories.

Veggie-Packed Quinoa Bowl

INGREDIENTS

- 1 cup quinoa, rinsed
- 2 cups vegetable broth
- 1 cup broccoli florets
- 1 cup cherry tomatoes, halved
- 1 red bell pepper, diced
- 1/2 cup grated carrot
- 1/4 cup sliced red onion
- 1 avocado, diced
- 1/4 cup fresh parsley, chopped
- 1/4 cup feta cheese, crumbled (optional)

For the Dressing:

- 3 tablespoons olive oil
- 2 tablespoons lemon juice
- 1 tablespoon balsamic vinegar
- 1 garlic clove, minced
- Salt and pepper to taste

DIRECTIONS

1. In a medium saucepan, bring the vegetable broth to a boil. Add the quinoa, reduce heat to low, cover, and simmer for about 15 minutes, or until the quinoa is cooked and the broth is absorbed. Fluff with a fork and let cool slightly.
2. While the quinoa is cooking, steam the broccoli florets until tender-crisp, about 3-4 minutes. Let cool.
3. In a large bowl, combine the cooked quinoa, steamed broccoli, cherry tomatoes, red bell pepper, grated carrot, red onion, avocado, parsley, and feta cheese if using.
4. In a small bowl, whisk together the dressing ingredients: olive oil, lemon juice, balsamic vinegar, minced garlic, salt, and pepper.
5. Pour the dressing over the quinoa and veggies, tossing to coat evenly.
6. Serve immediately or refrigerate until ready to eat.

Prep Time: 20 minutes
Cooking Time: 15 minutes
Servings: 4

Why I Recommend This Recipe: Veggie-Packed Quinoa Bowl is a nutrient-dense, balanced meal that's full of colorful vegetables, protein-rich quinoa, and healthy fats from avocado. It's an easy-to-make, satisfying lunch that supports weight loss and keeps you energized throughout the day.

DINNER DELIGHTS

Lemon Herb Baked Cod with Asparagus

INGREDIENTS

- 4 cod fillets (about 6 ounces each)
- 2 tablespoons olive oil
- 2 tablespoons fresh lemon juice
- 2 garlic cloves, minced
- 1 teaspoon dried oregano
- 1 teaspoon dried thyme
- Salt and pepper to taste
- 1 pound asparagus, trimmed
- 1 lemon, sliced

DIRECTIONS

1. Preheat your oven to 400°F (200°C). Line a baking sheet with parchment paper or lightly grease it.
2. In a small bowl, mix together the olive oil, lemon juice, minced garlic, oregano, thyme, salt, and pepper.
3. Place the cod fillets on one side of the prepared baking sheet. Brush the fillets with the lemon herb mixture.
4. Arrange the asparagus on the other side of the baking sheet. Drizzle with a little olive oil and season with salt and pepper.
5. Place lemon slices on top of the cod fillets.
6. Bake for 15-20 minutes, or until the cod is cooked through and flakes easily with a fork, and the asparagus is tender.
7. Serve immediately, garnished with additional lemon slices if desired.

Prep Time: 10 minutes
Cooking Time: 15-20 minutes
Servings: 4

Why I Recommend This Recipe: Lemon Herb Baked Cod with Asparagus is a light and flavorful dinner option that's rich in lean protein and packed with vitamins and minerals from the asparagus. This dish is easy to prepare and fits perfectly into a no-point weight loss plan, making it a delicious and nutritious choice for a satisfying meal.

Spaghetti Squash with Tomato Basil Sauce

INGREDIENTS

- 1 large spaghetti squash
- 2 tablespoons olive oil
- Salt and pepper to taste
- 1 onion, chopped
- 3 garlic cloves, minced
- 1 can (28 oz) crushed tomatoes
- 1/4 cup tomato paste
- 1 teaspoon dried oregano
- 1 teaspoon dried basil
- 1/4 teaspoon red pepper flakes (optional)
- 1/4 cup fresh basil, chopped
- 1/4 cup grated Parmesan cheese (optional)

DIRECTIONS

1. Preheat your oven to 375°F (190°C). Line a baking sheet with parchment paper.
2. Cut the spaghetti squash in half lengthwise and scoop out the seeds. Drizzle with 1 tablespoon of olive oil and season with salt and pepper. Place the squash halves cut side down on the prepared baking sheet.
3. Bake for 40-45 minutes, or until the squash is tender and can be easily shredded with a fork.
4. While the squash is baking, heat the remaining 1 tablespoon of olive oil in a large skillet over medium heat. Add the chopped onion and cook until softened, about 5 minutes.
5. Add the minced garlic and cook for another minute until fragrant.
6. Stir in the crushed tomatoes, tomato paste, dried oregano, dried basil, red pepper flakes (if using), salt, and pepper. Bring the sauce to a simmer and cook for 15-20 minutes, stirring occasionally.
7. Once the squash is done, use a fork to scrape out the strands of spaghetti squash into a large bowl.
8. Pour the tomato basil sauce over the spaghetti squash and toss to combine.
9. Serve immediately, topped with fresh basil and grated Parmesan cheese if desired.

Prep Time: 15 minutes
Cooking Time: 45 minutes
Servings: 4

Why I Recommend This Recipe: Spaghetti Squash with Tomato Basil Sauce is a hearty and satisfying dinner that's low in carbs and calories. The spaghetti squash is a great alternative to traditional pasta, and the homemade tomato basil sauce is rich in flavor and nutrients. This dish is perfect for those looking to enjoy a comforting meal without worrying about points or calories.

One-Pan Balsamic Chicken and Vegetables

INGREDIENTS

- 4 boneless, skinless chicken breasts
- 2 tablespoons olive oil
- 1/4 cup balsamic vinegar
- 1 tablespoon Dijon mustard
- 2 garlic cloves, minced
- 1 teaspoon dried basil
- 1 teaspoon dried oregano
- Salt and pepper to taste
- 1 cup cherry tomatoes, halved
- 1 red bell pepper, sliced
- 1 yellow bell pepper, sliced
- 1 zucchini, sliced into rounds
- 1 red onion, cut into wedges

DIRECTIONS

1. Preheat your oven to 400°F (200°C). Line a baking sheet with parchment paper or lightly grease it.
2. In a small bowl, whisk together the olive oil, balsamic vinegar, Dijon mustard, minced garlic, dried basil, dried oregano, salt, and pepper.
3. Place the chicken breasts on the prepared baking sheet and brush them with half of the balsamic mixture.
4. Arrange the cherry tomatoes, bell peppers, zucchini, and red onion around the chicken on the baking sheet. Drizzle the vegetables with the remaining balsamic mixture and toss to coat evenly.
5. Bake for 25-30 minutes, or until the chicken is cooked through and the vegetables are tender.
6. Serve immediately.

Prep Time: 15 minutes
Cooking Time: 25-30 minutes
Servings: 4

Why I Recommend This Recipe: One-Pan Balsamic Chicken and Vegetables is an easy and convenient dinner option that's full of flavor and packed with nutrients. The balsamic marinade adds a delicious tangy taste to both the chicken and vegetables, making this dish a healthy and satisfying meal that fits perfectly into a no-point weight loss plan.

Lentil and Vegetable Stir-Fry

INGREDIENTS

- 1 cup dry lentils, rinsed
- 2 cups vegetable broth
- 1 tablespoon olive oil
- 1 onion, sliced
- 2 garlic cloves, minced
- 1 red bell pepper, sliced
- 1 yellow bell pepper, sliced
- 1 zucchini, sliced into rounds
- 1 cup snap peas
- 1 cup broccoli florets
- 3 tablespoons low-sodium soy sauce
- 1 tablespoon rice vinegar
- 1 teaspoon sesame oil
- 1/4 cup chopped green onions
- 1 tablespoon sesame seeds (optional)

DIRECTIONS

1. In a medium saucepan, combine the lentils and vegetable broth. Bring to a boil, then reduce heat and simmer for about 20-25 minutes, or until the lentils are tender. Drain any excess liquid and set aside.

2. In a large skillet or wok, heat the olive oil over medium-high heat. Add the sliced onion and minced garlic, and cook until softened, about 3 minutes.

3. Add the red bell pepper, yellow bell pepper, zucchini, snap peas, and broccoli florets to the skillet. Stir-fry for about 5-7 minutes, or until the vegetables are tender-crisp.

4. In a small bowl, mix together the soy sauce, rice vinegar, and sesame oil.

5. Add the cooked lentils to the skillet with the vegetables. Pour the soy sauce mixture over the top and toss to coat everything evenly.

6. Cook for an additional 2-3 minutes, until everything is heated through.

7. Serve immediately, garnished with chopped green onions and sesame seeds if desired.

Prep Time: 15 minutes
Cooking Time: 25-30 minutes
Servings: 4

Why I Recommend This Recipe: Lentil and Vegetable Stir-Fry is a nutrient-rich, plant-based dinner that's high in protein and fiber. The colorful array of vegetables combined with hearty lentils makes this stir-fry both delicious and satisfying. It's a great way to enjoy a filling meal that aligns with your no-point weight loss goals.

DESSERTS

Chocolate Avocado Mousse

INGREDIENTS

- 2 ripe avocados, peeled and pitted
- 1/4 cup unsweetened cocoa powder
- 1/4 cup maple syrup
- 1/4 cup almond milk (or any milk of choice)
- 1 teaspoon vanilla extract
- Pinch of salt
- Fresh berries and mint leaves, for garnish (optional)

DIRECTIONS

1. In a food processor or blender, combine the avocados, cocoa powder, maple syrup, almond milk, vanilla extract, and a pinch of salt.
2. Blend until smooth and creamy, scraping down the sides as needed.
3. Taste and adjust sweetness if necessary, adding more maple syrup to your preference.
4. Spoon the mousse into serving dishes and chill in the refrigerator for at least 1 hour to set.
5. Before serving, garnish with fresh berries and mint leaves if desired.

Prep Time: 10 minutes
Chill Time: 1 hour
Servings: 4

Why I Recommend This Recipe: Chocolate Avocado Mousse is a rich and creamy dessert that's both decadent and healthy. The avocados provide healthy fats and a smooth texture, while the cocoa powder offers a rich chocolate flavor without the need for excessive sugar. This dessert is perfect for satisfying your sweet tooth while staying on track with your weight loss goals.

Baked Cinnamon Apples

INGREDIENTS

- 4 large apples (such as Honeycrisp or Granny Smith), cored
- 1/4 cup chopped walnuts
- 1/4 cup raisins
- 2 tablespoons maple syrup
- 1 teaspoon ground cinnamon
- 1/4 teaspoon ground nutmeg
- 1/4 cup water
- Optional: Greek yogurt or a dollop of whipped coconut cream, for serving

DIRECTIONS

1. Preheat your oven to 375°F (190°C). Place the cored apples in a baking dish.
2. In a small bowl, combine the chopped walnuts, raisins, maple syrup, ground cinnamon, and ground nutmeg.
3. Stuff the center of each apple with the walnut-raisin mixture.
4. Pour the water into the bottom of the baking dish to help steam the apples.
5. Cover the baking dish with aluminum foil and bake for 20 minutes. Remove the foil and bake for an additional 20-25 minutes, or until the apples are tender and easily pierced with a fork.
6. Serve the baked apples warm, optionally topped with a spoonful of Greek yogurt or whipped coconut cream.

Prep Time: 10 minutes
Cooking Time: 40-45 minutes
Servings: 4

Why I Recommend This Recipe: Baked Cinnamon Apples are a warm and comforting dessert that's naturally sweet and satisfying. The combination of baked apples, walnuts, and raisins creates a deliciously textured treat that's rich in fiber and healthy fats. This dessert is an excellent way to indulge in something sweet without compromising your weight loss journey.

Berry Chia Pudding

INGREDIENTS

- 1/4 cup chia seeds
- 1 cup unsweetened almond milk (or any milk of choice)
- 2 tablespoons maple syrup or honey
- 1 teaspoon vanilla extract
- 1 cup mixed berries (such as strawberries, blueberries, raspberries)
- Fresh mint leaves, for garnish (optional)

DIRECTIONS

Instructions:

1. In a medium bowl, combine the chia seeds, almond milk, maple syrup, and vanilla extract. Stir well to ensure the chia seeds are evenly distributed.

2. Cover and refrigerate for at least 4 hours or overnight, until the mixture thickens to a pudding-like consistency. Stir once or twice during this time to prevent clumping.

3. Before serving, gently mix the chia pudding again. Divide into serving bowls or jars.

4. Top with mixed berries and garnish with fresh mint leaves if desired.

Prep Time: 5 minutes
Chill Time: 4 hours (or overnight)
Servings: 4

Why I Recommend This Recipe: Berry Chia Pudding is a light and refreshing dessert that's rich in omega-3 fatty acids, fiber, and antioxidants. The chia seeds create a creamy, satisfying texture without the need for heavy creams or sugars, making this a perfect no-point dessert option for those on a weight loss journey.

Coconut Lime Energy Bites

INGREDIENTS

- 1 cup unsweetened shredded coconut
- 1/2 cup almond flour
- 1/4 cup honey or maple syrup
- 1/4 cup coconut oil, melted
- Zest of 1 lime
- Juice of 1 lime
- 1 teaspoon vanilla extract
- Pinch of salt

DIRECTIONS

1. In a large bowl, combine the shredded coconut, almond flour, honey, melted coconut oil, lime zest, lime juice, vanilla extract, and a pinch of salt.

2. Mix until the ingredients are well combined and a dough forms.

3. Using your hands, roll the mixture into small bite-sized balls.

4. Place the energy bites on a baking sheet lined with parchment paper and refrigerate for at least 30 minutes, until firm.

5. Store in an airtight container in the refrigerator for up to a week.

Prep Time: 10 minutes
Chill Time: 30 minutes
Servings: 12-15 bites

Why I Recommend This Recipe: Coconut Lime Energy Bites are a quick and easy dessert that packs a punch of flavor and nutrition. These bites are perfect for a sweet treat that's also full of healthy fats and fiber. They're great for curbing cravings and providing a quick energy boost without the need for refined sugars or empty calories.

Baked Pears with Walnuts and Honey

INGREDIENTS

- 4 ripe pears, halved and cored
- 1/4 cup chopped walnuts
- 2 tablespoons honey
- 1 teaspoon ground cinnamon
- 1/4 teaspoon ground nutmeg
- 1/4 cup water
- Optional: Greek yogurt or whipped coconut cream, for serving

DIRECTIONS

1. Preheat your oven to 375°F (190°C). Place the pear halves in a baking dish, cut side up.
2. In a small bowl, mix together the chopped walnuts, honey, ground cinnamon, and ground nutmeg.
3. Spoon the walnut mixture into the hollowed-out centers of the pears.
4. Pour the water into the bottom of the baking dish to help steam the pears.
5. Cover the baking dish with aluminum foil and bake for 20 minutes. Remove the foil and bake for an additional 15-20 minutes, or until the pears are tender and easily pierced with a fork.
6. Serve the baked pears warm, optionally topped with a dollop of Greek yogurt or whipped coconut cream.

Prep Time: 10 minutes
Cooking Time: 35-40 minutes
Servings: 4

Why I Recommend This Recipe: Baked Pears with Walnuts and Honey is a naturally sweet and wholesome dessert. The pears become soft and caramelized while the walnuts add a delightful crunch. This dessert is simple, elegant, and perfectly aligns with a no-point approach, making it a guilt-free treat.

Frozen Banana Bites

INGREDIENTS

- 2 large bananas, sliced into rounds
- 1/2 cup dark chocolate chips
- 1 tablespoon coconut oil
- 1/4 cup chopped nuts (such as almonds, peanuts, or walnuts)
- 1/4 cup unsweetened shredded coconut (optional)

DIRECTIONS

1. Line a baking sheet with parchment paper. Place the banana slices on the baking sheet and freeze for at least 1 hour, or until firm.

2. In a microwave-safe bowl, combine the dark chocolate chips and coconut oil. Microwave in 20-second intervals, stirring after each, until melted and smooth.

3. Dip each frozen banana slice halfway into the melted chocolate, then immediately sprinkle with chopped nuts and shredded coconut if desired.

4. Return the chocolate-dipped banana slices to the baking sheet and freeze for another 15-20 minutes, or until the chocolate is set.

5. Store the frozen banana bites in an airtight container in the freezer for up to 2 weeks.

Prep Time: 10 minutes
Chill Time: 1 hour 20 minutes

Why I Recommend This Recipe: Frozen Banana Bites are a refreshing and satisfying dessert that's easy to make and enjoy. The combination of creamy banana, rich dark chocolate, and crunchy nuts provides a delightful mix of textures and flavors. This no-point treat is perfect for cooling down on a warm day while staying aligned with your weight loss goals.

Green Detox Smoothie

INGREDIENTS

- 1 cup unsweetened almond milk (or any milk of choice)
- 1 cup fresh spinach leaves
- 1/2 cup frozen mango chunks
- 1/2 cup frozen pineapple chunks
- 1 ripe banana
- 1 tablespoon chia seeds
- 1 teaspoon grated ginger (optional)
- Juice of 1/2 lemon

DIRECTIONS

1. Add the almond milk, spinach, mango, pineapple, banana, chia seeds, ginger, and lemon juice to a blender.
2. Blend on high until smooth and creamy, scraping down the sides as needed.
3. Pour into a glass and serve immediately.

Prep Time: 5 minutes
Servings: 1

Why I Recommend This Recipe: The Green Detox Smoothie is a nutrient-packed beverage that's perfect for starting your day or enjoying as a mid-day refresher. The combination of leafy greens, tropical fruits, and chia seeds provides a boost of vitamins, minerals, and fiber. It's a delicious and easy way to support your weight loss journey and overall health.

Iced Herbal Tea with Citrus

INGREDIENTS

- 4 cups water
- 4 herbal tea bags (such as chamomile, mint, or hibiscus)
- 1 orange, sliced
- 1 lemon, sliced
- 1 lime, sliced
- 1 tablespoon honey or maple syrup (optional)
- Fresh mint leaves, for garnish
- Ice cubes

DIRECTIONS

1. Bring the water to a boil in a medium saucepan. Remove from heat and add the herbal tea bags.
2. Let the tea steep for 5-7 minutes, then remove the tea bags and let the tea cool to room temperature.
3. In a large pitcher, combine the cooled tea, orange slices, lemon slices, lime slices, and honey or maple syrup if using. Stir well.
4. Refrigerate for at least 1 hour to allow the flavors to meld.
5. To serve, fill glasses with ice cubes and pour the iced herbal tea over the top. Garnish with fresh mint leaves.

Prep Time: 10 minutes
Chill Time: 1 hour
Servings: 4

Why I Recommend This Recipe: Iced Herbal Tea with Citrus is a refreshing and hydrating beverage that's perfect for any time of the day. The blend of citrus fruits adds a natural sweetness and a burst of vitamin C, while the herbal tea offers calming and soothing properties. This beverage is low in calories and can be enjoyed guilt-free, aligning perfectly with a no-point weight loss plan.

Cucumber Mint Infused Water

INGREDIENTS

- 1 large cucumber, thinly sliced
- 1/4 cup fresh mint leaves
- 1 lemon, thinly sliced
- 8 cups water
- Ice cubes

DIRECTIONS

1. In a large pitcher, combine the cucumber slices, mint leaves, and lemon slices.
2. Pour the water over the ingredients and stir gently.
3. Refrigerate for at least 2 hours to allow the flavors to infuse.
4. Serve over ice cubes in glasses, garnished with additional cucumber slices or mint leaves if desired.

Prep Time: 10 minutes
Infuse Time: 2 hours
Servings: 8

Why I Recommend This Recipe: Cucumber Mint Infused Water is a refreshing and hydrating drink that's perfect for staying cool and hydrated. The cucumber and mint provide a light, crisp flavor, while the lemon adds a zesty touch. This beverage is a great way to increase your water intake without any added calories, supporting your weight loss goals effortlessly.

Almond Joy Smoothie

INGREDIENTS

- 1 cup unsweetened almond milk
- 1 banana
- 1 tablespoon unsweetened cocoa powder
- 1 tablespoon almond butter
- 1 tablespoon unsweetened shredded coconut
- 1 teaspoon vanilla extract
- Ice cubes

DIRECTIONS

Instructions:

1. Add the almond milk, banana, cocoa powder, almond butter, shredded coconut, vanilla extract, and a handful of ice cubes to a blender.
2. Blend on high until smooth and creamy, scraping down the sides as needed.
3. Pour into a glass and serve immediately, optionally topped with a sprinkle of shredded coconut.

Prep Time: 5 minutes
Servings: 1

Why I Recommend This Recipe: The Almond Joy Smoothie is a delicious and indulgent beverage that tastes like a treat but is packed with healthy ingredients. The combination of almond butter, cocoa powder, and coconut provides a satisfying flavor reminiscent of the classic candy bar, but without the added sugars and unhealthy fats. This smoothie is perfect for a nutritious snack or even a light meal replacement that

Turmeric Ginger Latte

INGREDIENTS

- 2 cups unsweetened almond milk (or any milk of choice)
- 1 teaspoon ground turmeric
- 1/2 teaspoon ground ginger
- 1/2 teaspoon ground cinnamon
- 1 tablespoon honey or maple syrup (optional)
- 1/2 teaspoon vanilla extract
- Pinch of black pepper
- Pinch of ground nutmeg (optional)
- Ice cubes (for iced version)

DIRECTIONS

1. In a small saucepan, heat the almond milk over medium heat until warm but not boiling.
2. Whisk in the turmeric, ginger, cinnamon, honey or maple syrup (if using), vanilla extract, and black pepper until well combined.
3. Continue to heat for about 5 minutes, stirring occasionally, until the mixture is hot and the spices are fully integrated.
4. Pour the latte into a mug and sprinkle with a pinch of ground nutmeg if desired.
5. For an iced version, let the mixture cool slightly and then pour over ice cubes.

Prep Time: 5 minutes
Cooking Time: 5 minutes
Servings: 2

Why I Recommend This Recipe: Turmeric Ginger Latte is a warming and soothing beverage known for its anti-inflammatory properties. The combination of turmeric and ginger supports digestion and overall wellness, making this latte a healthy choice. It's a delicious and nutritious way to enjoy a no-point drink that fits perfectly into your weight loss plan.

Watermelon Basil Cooler

INGREDIENTS

- 4 cups watermelon, cubed and seeds removed
- 1/4 cup fresh basil leaves
- Juice of 1 lime
- 1 cup cold water
- Ice cubes

DIRECTIONS

1. In a blender, combine the watermelon cubes, basil leaves, lime juice, and cold water.
2. Blend on high until smooth and well combined.
3. Pour the mixture through a fine-mesh strainer into a pitcher to remove any pulp, if desired.
4. Serve over ice cubes in glasses, garnished with additional basil leaves and lime slices if desired.

Prep Time: 10 minutes
Servings: 4

Why I Recommend This Recipe: Watermelon Basil Cooler is a refreshing and hydrating beverage that's perfect for hot days. The watermelon provides natural sweetness and hydration, while the basil adds a unique, aromatic flavor. This cooler is low in calories and high in vitamins, making it an ideal no-point beverage for those looking to stay healthy and refreshed.

Meal Plans and Tips

Two-Week No Point Meal Plan

This two-week meal plan features a variety of delicious and nutritious no-point recipes. It includes breakfast, lunch, dinner, and snacks to keep you satisfied and energized throughout the day. Each recipe aligns with the goal of helping you gain energy and lose weight without the need to count calories.

Week 1

Monday

- **Breakfast:** Greek Yogurt Parfait with Mixed Berries and Chia Seeds
- **Lunch:** Lentil and Vegetable Stir-Fry
- **Dinner:** One-Pan Balsamic Chicken and Vegetables
- **Snacks:** Carrot and Hummus Bites, Apple Slices with Almond Butter

Tuesday

- **Breakfast:** Overnight Oats with Almond Butter and Banana
- **Lunch:** Quinoa and Black Bean Salad
- **Dinner:** Lemon Herb Grilled Salmon with Steamed Asparagus
- **Snacks:** Cucumber Mint Infused Water, Mixed Nuts

Wednesday

- **Breakfast:** Spinach and Feta Omelette
- **Lunch:** Chicken and Avocado Salad

- **Dinner:** Zucchini Noodles with Pesto and Cherry Tomatoes
- **Snacks:** Berry Chia Pudding, Fresh Strawberries

Thursday

- **Breakfast:** Blueberry Almond Smoothie
- **Lunch:** Greek Chickpea Salad
- **Dinner:** Baked Lemon Garlic Cod with Roasted Brussels Sprouts
- **Snacks:** Carrot Sticks with Guacamole, Frozen Banana Bites

Friday

- **Breakfast:** Veggie Breakfast Burrito
- **Lunch:** Tuna Salad Lettuce Wraps
- **Dinner:** Spaghetti Squash with Marinara Sauce and Turkey Meatballs
- **Snacks:** Apple Cinnamon Energy Bites, Celery Sticks with Peanut Butter

Saturday

- **Breakfast:** Avocado Toast with Poached Eggs
- **Lunch:** Quinoa Tabbouleh
- **Dinner:** Chicken and Vegetable Stir-Fry
- **Snacks:** Watermelon Basil Cooler, Mixed Berries

Sunday

- **Breakfast:** Chocolate Avocado Mousse (as a treat)

- **Lunch:** Spinach and Strawberry Salad with Balsamic Vinaigrette
- **Dinner:** Grilled Chicken with Quinoa and Steamed Broccoli
- **Snacks:** Turmeric Ginger Latte, Almond Joy Smoothie

Week 2

Monday

- **Breakfast:** Berry Green Smoothie
- **Lunch:** Mediterranean Couscous Salad
- **Dinner:** Stuffed Bell Peppers with Ground Turkey and Vegetables
- **Snacks:** Almond Joy Smoothie, Fresh Carrot Sticks

Tuesday

- **Breakfast:** Mango Coconut Chia Pudding
- **Lunch:** Lentil Soup with Spinach
- **Dinner:** Shrimp and Zucchini Noodles with Garlic Sauce
- **Snacks:** Greek Yogurt with Honey and Walnuts, Cucumber Slices

Wednesday

- **Breakfast:** Apple Cinnamon Overnight Oats
- **Lunch:** Grilled Chicken Caesar Salad (without croutons)
- **Dinner:** Baked Salmon with Quinoa and Steamed Green Beans
- **Snacks:** Berry Chia Pudding, Fresh Pineapple Chunks

Thursday

- **Breakfast:** Spinach and Mushroom Frittata
- **Lunch:** Avocado and Black Bean Salad
- **Dinner:** Grilled Shrimp Skewers with Mixed Vegetables
- **Snacks:** Almond Joy Smoothie, Sliced Bell Peppers with Hummus

Friday

- **Breakfast:** Peach and Almond Smoothie
- **Lunch:** Turkey and Veggie Lettuce Wraps
- **Dinner:** Lemon Rosemary Chicken with Roasted Sweet Potatoes
- **Snacks:** Apple Slices with Almond Butter, Mixed Nuts

Saturday

- **Breakfast:** Greek Yogurt Parfait with Granola and Blueberries
- **Lunch:** Quinoa and Black Bean Salad
- **Dinner:** Beef and Broccoli Stir-Fry with Brown Rice
- **Snacks:** Coconut Lime Energy Bites, Fresh Grapes

Sunday

- **Breakfast:** Banana Oat Pancakes
- **Lunch:** Spinach and Feta Stuffed Portobello Mushrooms
- **Dinner:** Grilled Chicken with Mango Salsa and Steamed Asparagus

- **Snacks:** Watermelon Basil Cooler, Mixed Berries

This meal plan includes a variety of meals that will keep your taste buds happy and help you lose weight. Each recipe is made to be healthy, tasty, and in line with the no-point theory. This way, you can enjoy your food without having to worry about how many calories it has.

Quick and Easy Meal Prep Tips

Meal prepping can be a game-changer for anyone looking to maintain a healthy diet without spending hours in the kitchen every day. By dedicating a bit of time each week to prepare your meals in advance, you can save time, reduce stress, and stay on track with your weight loss goals. Here are some quick and easy meal prep tips to help you get started:

1. Plan Your Meals

- **Weekly Menu:** Create a weekly menu that outlines your meals for breakfast, lunch, dinner, and snacks. This helps you stay organized and ensures you have a variety of meals to enjoy.

- **Grocery List:** Based on your menu, make a detailed grocery list. This will save you time at the store and ensure you have all the ingredients you need.

2. Batch Cooking

- **Cook in Bulk:** Prepare large batches of staple ingredients like grains (quinoa, rice), proteins (chicken, beans), and roasted vegetables. Store them in the fridge or freezer for easy assembly throughout the week.

- **One-Pot Meals:** Utilize recipes that can be made in one pot or one pan, such as soups, stews, and casseroles. They save time on cooking and cleaning.

3. Use Versatile Ingredients

- **Mix and Match:** Choose ingredients that can be used in multiple dishes. For example, roasted chicken can be used in salads, wraps, and stir-fries.

- **Flavor Variations:** Keep a variety of spices and sauces on hand to quickly change up the flavor profile of your meals without needing to cook something entirely new.

4. Invest in Good Containers

- **Storage Solutions:** Use high-quality, BPA-free containers that are microwave and dishwasher safe. Clear containers make it easy to see what's inside, and uniform sizes help with organization.

- **Portion Control:** Pre-portion your meals into individual servings. This helps with portion control and makes it easy to grab a meal on the go.

5. Prep Snacks and Breakfasts

- **Easy Breakfasts:** Prepare quick breakfast options like overnight oats, chia pudding, or smoothie packs that you can just blend in the morning.

- **Healthy Snacks:** Keep healthy snacks like cut veggies, hummus, nuts, and fruit readily available. Pre-portioning these snacks can help you avoid unhealthy choices.

6. Use Your Freezer Wisely

- **Freeze Portions:** Freeze individual portions of soups, stews, and casseroles. They can be reheated quickly for a nutritious meal when you're short on time.
- **Frozen Fruits and Vegetables:** Keep a stash of frozen fruits and vegetables. They're just as nutritious as fresh and can be easily added to smoothies, stir-fries, and more.

7. Make It a Routine

- **Set a Schedule:** Dedicate a specific day and time each week for meal prep. Consistency helps turn meal prep into a habit.
- **Involve the Family:** Get your family involved in meal prep. It can be a fun activity and also teaches valuable cooking skills.

8. Simplify Recipes

- **Quick Recipes:** Choose recipes with fewer ingredients and steps. Simple recipes are easier to prepare and often just as delicious.
- **Time-Saving Tools:** Use kitchen tools like a slow cooker, Instant Pot, or food processor to cut down on prep and cooking time.

9. Label Everything

- **Date and Contents:** Label your containers with the date and contents. This helps you keep track of what needs to be eaten first and prevents food waste.

- **Meal Categories:** Consider color-coding labels for different meal categories (e.g., green for veggies, blue for proteins) to quickly identify what you need.

10. Stay Flexible

- **Adjust as Needed:** Your meal plan doesn't have to be rigid. Be flexible and adjust based on your schedule, cravings, and what you have on hand.

- **Leftovers:** Don't be afraid to repurpose leftovers into new meals. For example, leftover roasted vegetables can be added to a frittata or salad.

If you follow these quick and easy tips for meal prep, you can enjoy a range of healthy, no-point meals with little work. Preparing meals ahead of time not only saves you time and stress, but it also helps you stick to your weight loss and health goals.

How to Customize Recipes for Dietary Needs

Customizing recipes to suit various dietary needs is essential for ensuring that everyone can enjoy nutritious and delicious meals. Whether you're accommodating allergies, intolerances, or specific dietary preferences, making adjustments to recipes can be simple and effective. Here's how you can tailor recipes to meet different dietary requirements without compromising on taste or nutrition.

1. Understanding Common Dietary Needs

- **Gluten-Free:** Avoids wheat, barley, rye, and other gluten-containing grains.
- **Dairy-Free:** Eliminates milk and milk products.
- **Vegetarian:** Excludes meat, poultry, and fish.
- **Vegan:** Excludes all animal products, including meat, dairy, eggs, and honey.
- **Low-Carb/Keto:** Focuses on reducing carbohydrate intake, emphasizing proteins and fats.
- **Nut-Free:** Avoids all nuts and nut-based products.
- **Paleo:** Emphasizes whole foods, avoiding processed foods, grains, dairy, and legumes.

2. Substituting Ingredients

Gluten-Free

- **Flours:** Replace wheat flour with gluten-free alternatives like almond flour, coconut flour, rice flour, or a gluten-free all-purpose flour blend.
- **Pasta:** Use gluten-free pasta made from rice, quinoa, or lentils.
- **Bread:** Substitute with gluten-free bread or make your own using gluten-free flour mixes.

Dairy-Free

- **Milk:** Swap cow's milk for plant-based alternatives like almond milk, soy milk, coconut milk, or oat milk.
- **Butter:** Use dairy-free butter substitutes, coconut oil, or olive oil.
- **Cheese:** Replace cheese with dairy-free cheese made from nuts, soy, or coconut, or use nutritional yeast for a cheesy flavor.

Vegetarian

- **Meat:** Replace meat with plant-based proteins like tofu, tempeh, seitan, legumes, lentils, and chickpeas.

- **Broth:** Use vegetable broth instead of chicken or beef broth.

Vegan

- **Eggs:** Use flaxseed meal or chia seeds mixed with water as an egg substitute (1 tablespoon of seeds + 3 tablespoons of water = 1 egg). Applesauce or mashed bananas can also work in baking.
- **Honey:** Substitute with maple syrup, agave nectar, or date syrup.
- **Gelatin:** Use agar-agar or pectin for vegan-friendly gelling agents.

Low-Carb/Keto

- **Grains:** Substitute grains with cauliflower rice, zucchini noodles, or shirataki noodles.
- **Sugar:** Use low-carb sweeteners like stevia, erythritol, or monk fruit sweetener.
- **Flours:** Replace regular flour with almond flour, coconut flour, or flaxseed meal.

Nut-Free

- **Nut Butters:** Use seed butters like sunflower seed butter or tahini.
- **Flours:** Substitute nut flours with oat flour, rice flour, or coconut flour.
- **Milk:** Use coconut milk or oat milk instead of almond milk or other nut milks.

3. Adjusting Cooking Methods

- **Baking:** Ensure gluten-free baked goods have a binding agent like xanthan gum or guar gum to mimic the elasticity of gluten.
- **Sautéing:** Use olive oil, coconut oil, or avocado oil instead of butter for dairy-free or vegan cooking.
- **Marinating:** For vegan options, marinate tofu or tempeh in flavorful sauces instead of meat.

4. Enhancing Flavor Without Additives

- **Herbs and Spices:** Use fresh herbs and spices to enhance flavor naturally. This is especially useful for low-sodium, low-fat, or heart-healthy diets.
- **Citrus:** Add lemon or lime juice for a burst of flavor without added calories or sodium.

5. Reading Labels and Choosing Products

- **Check Ingredients:** Always read food labels to ensure there are no hidden allergens or animal products.
- **Certified Products:** Look for certified gluten-free, organic, or non-GMO labels if they align with your dietary needs.

6. Keeping Nutrition Balanced

- **Protein:** Ensure adequate protein intake by incorporating beans, lentils, tofu, tempeh, quinoa, and nuts/seeds (if not allergic).
- **Fiber:** Include plenty of fruits, vegetables, and whole grains (if allowed) to maintain fiber intake.
- **Healthy Fats:** Use sources of healthy fats like avocado, nuts/seeds (if not allergic), and olive oil.

7. Customizing for Taste Preferences

- **Spiciness:** Adjust the level of spices and seasonings to cater to personal heat tolerance.
- **Sweetness:** Modify sweeteners to suit taste, using natural options like fruit purees or dates.

8. Making it Kid-Friendly

- **Texture:** Consider softer textures and milder flavors for children's meals.
- **Presentation:** Make meals fun with colorful vegetables and creative presentations to encourage kids to eat healthy.

Made in the USA
Las Vegas, NV
02 July 2024